Keto Diet for Women Over 50

A Beginner's 3-Week Step-by-Step Guide with Curated Recipes and a Meal Plan

mf

copyright © 2020 Stephanie Hinderock

All rights reserved No part of this book may be reproduced, or stored in a retrieval system, or transmitted in any form or by any means, electronic, mechanical, photocopying, recording, or otherwise, without express written permission of the publisher.

Disclaimer

By reading this disclaimer, you are accepting the terms of the disclaimer in full. If you disagree with this disclaimer, please do not read the guide.

All of the content within this guide is provided for informational and educational purposes only, and should not be accepted as independent medical or other professional advice. The author is not a doctor, physician, nurse, mental health provider, or registered nutritionist/dietician. Therefore, using and reading this guide does not establish any form of a physician-patient relationship.

Always consult with a physician or another qualified health provider with any issues or questions you might have regarding any sort of medical condition. Do not ever disregard any qualified professional medical advice or delay seeking that advice because of anything you have read in this guide. The information in this guide is not intended to be any sort of medical advice and should not be used in lieu of any medical advice by a licensed and qualified medical professional.

The information in this guide has been compiled from a variety of known sources. However, the author cannot attest to or guarantee the accuracy of each source and thus should not be held liable for any errors or omissions.

You acknowledge that the publisher of this guide will not be held liable for any loss or damage of any kind incurred as a result of this guide or the reliance on any information provided within this guide. You acknowledge and agree that you assume all risk and responsibility for any action you undertake in response to the information in this guide.

Using this guide does not guarantee any particular result (e.g., weight loss or a cure). By reading this guide, you acknowledge that there are no guarantees to any specific outcome or results you can expect.

All product names, diet plans, or names used in this guide are for identification purposes only and are the property of their respective owners. The use of these names does not imply endorsement. All other trademarks cited herein are the property of their respective owners.

Where applicable, this guide is not intended to be a substitute for the original work of this diet plan and is, at most, a supplement to the original work for this diet plan and never a direct substitute. This guide is a personal expression of the facts of that diet plan.

Where applicable, persons shown in the cover images are stock photography models and the publisher has obtained the rights to use the images through license agreements with third-party stock image companies.

Table of Contents

Introduction — 7
The Ketogenic Diet — 10
    Understanding Ketosis — 10
    Composition of a Healthy Ketogenic Diet — 11
    How Does Keto Affect Women Over 50? — 12
    Principles of the Ketogenic Diet for Women Over 50 — 19
    Disadvantages of the Ketogenic Diet — 21
The Types of Ketogenic Diet — 23
    Standard Ketogenic Diet (SKD) — 23
    Targeted Keto Diet (TKD) — 24
    Cyclical Keto Diet (CKD) — 24
    High Protein Keto Diet (HPKD) — 25
How Do You Get Started? — 26
    Step 1: Do Your Research — 26
    Step 2: Plan Your Diet Thoroughly — 27
    Step 3: Make Your Cupboards and Refrigerator Keto-Friendly — 30
    Step 4: Equip Yourself with Helpful Tools — 33
    Step 5: Prepare Yourself — 36
    Foods to Eat in the Ketogenic Diet for Women Over 50 — 39
    Foods to Avoid in the Ketogenic Diet for Women Over 50 — 42
Favorite Keto Meal Plans and Recipes — 45
    7-Day Sample Meal Plan — 45
Sample Recipes — 49
    Cauliflower Pizza — 50
    Steak and Mushrooms — 52
    Ketogenic Pizza — 54
    Keto Pesto Chicken — 56
    Mushroom Omelet — 58

Sesame Chicken	59
Mexican Style Beef Chili	61
Western Omelet	63
Grilled Lamb	65
Roasted Veggies	67
Ground Beef Stroganoff	69
Banana Bread	71
Zero Carb Buttery Noodles	73
Zero Carb Bread	74
Baked Turkey Wings	75
Conclusion	**77**
FAQs for the Ketogenic Diet for Women Over 50	**81**
References	**84**

Introduction

Navigating the maze of nutrition and dieting can be particularly challenging for women over 50. With changes in metabolism, hormone levels, and overall body composition, finding a diet that effectively supports health and weight management is crucial. Among the myriad of dietary approaches available today, the ketogenic diet stands out for its potential benefits, especially for women in this age group.

Feeling more energetic, maintaining a healthy weight, and reducing the risks of chronic diseases—all achievable through dietary changes. This isn't just wishful thinking; it's a realistic outcome for many who have embraced the ketogenic (keto) diet. But what exactly is the keto diet, and why is it particularly beneficial for women over 50?

The keto diet is a low-carbohydrate, high-fat eating plan designed to shift the body's metabolism from relying on glucose for energy to burning fats instead. This metabolic state, known as ketosis, can offer remarkable health benefits. For women over 50, transitioning to a keto lifestyle can address common issues such as weight gain, declining energy levels, and increased risk of diabetes and cardiovascular diseases.

Understanding why the keto diet is effective begins with a brief look at how it works. By drastically reducing carbohydrate intake and replacing it with healthy fats, the body is prompted to use fat as its primary energy source. This process not only helps in burning stored fat but also stabilizes blood sugar levels, which is crucial for women experiencing insulin resistance or metabolic syndrome.

Waking up each day with sustained energy, fewer hunger pangs, and improved mental clarity—these are just some of the benefits reported by women over 50 who have successfully adopted the keto diet. Additionally, this dietary approach can lead to significant weight loss, making it easier to manage menopause-related weight gain. Beyond the scale, the keto diet has shown promise in enhancing overall health by reducing inflammation, lowering cholesterol levels, and improving heart health.

Hormonal balance is another critical area where the keto diet excels. As women age, hormonal fluctuations can lead to a variety of health concerns, including weight gain, mood swings, and decreased bone density. The keto diet's emphasis on healthy fats can aid in hormone production and regulation, offering a natural way to mitigate these issues.

In this guide, you will discover;

- What is a Ketogenic Diet?
- The Types of Ketogenic Diet
- How Does Keto Affect Women Over 50?
- How Do You Get Started with The Ketogenic Diet?
- Favorite Keto Meal Plans and Recipes

Embarking on a keto journey may seem daunting, but this comprehensive guide is here to make the transition smooth and manageable. It covers everything from the basic principles of the keto diet to practical tips for meal planning and overcoming common challenges. By following this guide, women over 50 can take charge of their health, experience the transformative power of the keto diet, and thrive in this empowering phase of life.

If you're ready to unlock the full potential of your golden years, dive into this guide and discover how the ketogenic diet can help you achieve lasting health and vitality.

The Ketogenic Diet

The Keto Diet, or ketogenic diet, is a nutritional regimen that significantly reduces carbohydrate intake while emphasizing high-quality dietary proteins and healthy fats. By drastically cutting down on carbohydrates, the body's glucose reserves are depleted, prompting a shift to a metabolic state known as ketosis.

Understanding Ketosis

Ketosis is a natural physiological process that kicks in when glucose levels in the body drop significantly. In this state, the liver breaks down fats to produce molecules called ketones, which then become the primary source of energy, replacing glucose. This alternative energy pathway allows vital organs, including the brain, to function efficiently by utilizing ketone bodies for their biological processes.

Measuring and maintaining ketosis is crucial for those on a ketogenic diet. This can be done through meticulous monitoring of ketone levels in the urine or blood. Concurrently, blood sugar and insulin levels typically decrease significantly, aligning with the dietary goals of the keto regimen.

Composition of a Healthy Ketogenic Diet

In a typical diet, carbohydrates constitute about 50% or more of daily caloric intake, with fats and proteins making up 30% and 15%, respectively. Unfortunately, much of the carbohydrate consumption comes from unhealthy sources like sweets, starches, and junk food, which can negatively impact health and weight.

In stark contrast, a ketogenic diet restricts carbohydrate intake to a maximum of 10% of total calories, sourced primarily from healthy choices such as green vegetables, legumes, and berries. Protein intake is moderately increased to 20%, encouraging the consumption of omega-3-rich fish and grass-fed meats like beef.

The cornerstone of the keto diet is its high-fat content, which makes up approximately 70% of daily caloric intake. However, it's vital to focus on consuming healthy fats. Unsaturated fats, both monounsaturated and polyunsaturated, offer numerous health benefits, including improved heart health and better cholesterol levels. Foods rich in these beneficial fats include avocados, nuts, seeds, coconut, and various oils.

How Does Keto Affect Women Over 50?

For women over 50, the ketogenic diet offers a host of potential benefits that go beyond weight loss. As the body undergoes significant changes with age, including hormonal shifts and a slower metabolism, adopting a keto lifestyle can support overall health and well-being in various ways. By significantly reducing carbohydrate intake and increasing healthy fats, the keto diet can help stabilize blood sugar levels, which is particularly important for those at risk of diabetes.

1. **Hormonal Balance**

    One of the most significant changes women experience after 50 is menopause, which brings about a dramatic shift in hormone levels. This life stage typically occurs between the ages of 45 and 55 and can last several years, leading to a range of symptoms. These symptoms can include weight gain, mood swings, hot flashes, night sweats, and decreased bone density. Menopause also increases the risk of developing osteoporosis and cardiovascular diseases due to the decline in estrogen levels.

    The ketogenic diet, with its emphasis on healthy fats, can help support hormone production and balance during this transition. Fats are essential for the synthesis of hormones, and consuming adequate amounts can help mitigate some of the uncomfortable symptoms associated with menopause. Healthy fats, like those found in avocados, nuts, seeds, and oily fish, provide the building blocks for hormone production. Additionally, the ketogenic diet may help stabilize blood sugar levels and reduce inflammation, further aiding in the management of menopausal symptoms.

By focusing on nutrient-dense foods and maintaining a balanced intake of fats, proteins, and carbohydrates, women can support their bodies through the hormonal changes of menopause and improve their overall well-being.

2. Metabolic Health

As women age, their metabolism tends to slow down, leading to weight gain and an increased risk of metabolic conditions like type 2 diabetes and metabolic syndrome. This metabolic decline can be attributed to a variety of factors, including hormonal changes, decreased muscle mass, and lifestyle choices.

The keto diet's low-carb, high-fat approach helps stabilize blood sugar levels and improve insulin sensitivity, which is crucial for metabolic health. By significantly reducing carbohydrate intake, the body enters a state of ketosis, where it relies more on fats for energy instead of glucose. This metabolic shift can assist in maintaining a healthier weight and reducing the risk of metabolic diseases. Moreover, the keto diet's emphasis on healthy fats and moderate protein intake can help preserve lean muscle mass, further supporting an efficient metabolism and overall well-being.

3. **Bone Health**

Postmenopausal women are at a higher risk of osteoporosis due to decreased estrogen levels, which play a crucial role in bone density maintenance. This hormonal change can lead to a faster rate of bone loss, making the bones more fragile and susceptible to fractures. While the keto diet itself is not specifically designed to enhance bone health, it encourages the consumption of nutrient-dense foods rich in vitamins and minerals essential for bone health, such as leafy greens, fatty fish, nuts, and seeds.

These foods provide important nutrients like calcium, magnesium, and vitamin D, which are vital for maintaining strong bones. Additionally, incorporating weight-bearing exercises alongside the keto diet can further support bone health by stimulating bone formation and reducing bone loss. Maintaining a healthy weight through the keto diet can also reduce the stress on bones and joints, thereby supporting overall skeletal health and potentially decreasing the risk of joint-related issues, such as arthritis.

4. **Cognitive Function**

Cognitive decline is a significant concern for many women as they age, impacting memory, attention, and overall brain function. The brain can utilize ketones more efficiently than glucose, and this alternative energy source has been shown to support cognitive function.

Some studies suggest that a ketogenic diet may offer neuroprotective benefits, potentially reducing the risk of neurodegenerative diseases like Alzheimer's and Parkinson's. By providing a steady supply of ketones, the keto diet can help maintain mental clarity, improve focus, and enhance overall cognitive performance.

Furthermore, ketones have been shown to have anti-inflammatory properties, which can contribute to brain health by reducing oxidative stress. Incorporating a ketogenic diet as part of a holistic approach to brain health could be a valuable strategy for women looking to preserve their cognitive abilities as they age.

5. **Weight Management**

   Weight gain is a common issue for women over 50 due to hormonal changes and a slower metabolism. As estrogen levels decline, the distribution of body fat changes, often leading to increased abdominal fat. The keto diet helps in weight management by promoting satiety and reducing hunger pangs.

   The high-fat, moderate-protein, and low-carb composition of the diet ensures that individuals feel fuller for longer periods, thereby decreasing overall calorie intake. This reduction in calorie consumption can lead to gradual weight loss and help stabilize weight over time.

   Additionally, the keto diet encourages the body to burn fat for energy, which can be particularly beneficial for postmenopausal women who find it challenging to maintain or lose weight through traditional dieting methods. By focusing on healthy fats and nutrient-dense foods, the keto diet also supports overall health, making it a sustainable option for long-term weight management.

6. **Heart Health**

   Cardiovascular health is a critical concern for aging women, as the risk of heart disease increases with age. This is due to various factors, including hormonal changes, increased blood pressure, and the accumulation of arterial plaque over time. The keto diet, when followed correctly, can have a positive impact on heart health. By reducing carbohydrate intake and focusing on healthy fats, the diet can help lower levels of bad cholesterol (LDL) and increase good cholesterol (HDL), which are crucial for maintaining a healthy cardiovascular system.

Additionally, the anti-inflammatory properties of the ketogenic diet can contribute to improved heart health by reducing the inflammation that can lead to heart disease. The diet promotes the consumption of anti-inflammatory foods and minimizes the intake of processed and sugary foods that can exacerbate inflammation.

However, it's important to choose the right types of fats, such as those found in avocados, nuts, seeds, and oily fish, to ensure cardiovascular benefits. Incorporating a variety of these healthy fats into your diet can provide essential nutrients and fatty acids that support heart function and overall well-being.

Moreover, staying hydrated and maintaining a balanced intake of electrolytes like sodium, potassium, and magnesium is vital for heart health, especially when following the keto diet. These minerals help regulate heart rhythm and blood pressure, contributing to a healthier heart.

Regular physical activity and avoiding sedentary habits can further enhance the benefits of the keto diet on cardiovascular health. By making these mindful choices, aging women can significantly reduce their risk of heart disease and enjoy a healthier, more vibrant life.

7. **Energy Levels**

Many women over 50 experience fluctuations in energy levels, often feeling fatigued and sluggish. These fluctuations can be due to various factors such as hormonal changes, slower metabolism, and lifestyle habits. The ketogenic diet can provide a more stable and sustained energy source compared to a high-carb diet. By burning fats for fuel, the body avoids the energy spikes and crashes associated with glucose metabolism.

This process, known as ketosis, helps maintain a steady supply of energy throughout the day. As a result, women on a ketogenic diet may experience enhanced overall energy levels, enabling them to stay active and engaged in their daily activities. This can also contribute to improved mood and better overall health, making it easier to enjoy hobbies, exercise, and social interactions.

The ketogenic diet offers a range of benefits that can address the unique health challenges faced by women over 50. From hormonal balance and metabolic health to cognitive function and heart health, the keto diet provides a holistic approach to aging gracefully. As with any dietary change, it's essential to consult with a healthcare provider to ensure that the ketogenic diet is appropriate for individual health needs and goals. By embracing the keto lifestyle, women over 50 can unlock a pathway to improved health, vitality, and wellness.

Principles of the Ketogenic Diet for Women Over 50

When considering the ketogenic diet for women over 50, it's essential to understand its underlying principles and guidelines. Here are some key principles to keep in mind when following a keto lifestyle:

1. **Low Carbohydrate Intake**: Limit carbohydrate consumption to 5-10% of daily calories to deplete glucose reserves and enter a state of ketosis.
2. **High Fat Consumption**: Consume 70-75% of daily calories from healthy fats such as avocados, nuts, seeds, olives, and fatty fish to support heart health and hormone production.

3. ***Moderate Protein Intake***: Ensure 15-20% of daily calories come from high-quality protein sources like grass-fed beef, poultry, eggs, and plant-based proteins to maintain muscle mass.
4. ***Nutrient-Dense Foods***: Focus on nutrient-rich foods like leafy greens, non-starchy vegetables, and berries to provide essential vitamins and minerals.
5. ***Hydration***: Drink plenty of water and electrolyte-rich beverages to maintain fluid balance and prevent dehydration often associated with low-carb intake.
6. ***Monitoring Ketone Levels***: Regularly measure ketone levels using urine strips, blood tests, or breath analyzers to ensure the body remains in ketosis.
7. ***Personalized Adjustments***: Adjust the diet based on individual health status, activity levels, and specific goals with the guidance of a dietitian or healthcare provider.
8. ***Balanced Meal Planning***: Plan meals to include appropriate portions of fats, proteins, and low-carb vegetables to ensure nutritional balance and variety.
9. ***Regular Physical Activity***: Combine the diet with strength training, cardio exercises, and flexibility workouts to enhance overall health and support metabolic function.
10. ***Mindful Eating***: Practice mindful eating to better manage dietary choices and recognize hunger and

satiety cues, promoting a healthier relationship with food.
11. ***Ongoing Health Monitoring***: Schedule regular check-ups to monitor the diet's impact on overall health, including blood tests for cholesterol levels, blood sugar, and other key markers.

By adhering to these principles, women over 50 can effectively harness the benefits of the ketogenic diet, promoting improved health, vitality, and quality of life.

Disadvantages of the Ketogenic Diet

While the ketogenic diet can be a beneficial dietary approach for women over 50, there are also some potential disadvantages to consider.

1. ***Limited Food Choices***: The restrictive nature of the diet may make it challenging to adhere to, as it eliminates many commonly consumed foods like grains, legumes, and fruits. This can result in feelings of deprivation and may lead to difficulty sustaining the diet long-term.
2. ***Potential Nutrient Deficiencies***: Eliminating certain food groups can increase the risk of nutrient deficiencies if not properly planned and monitored. Specifically, deficiencies in fiber, magnesium, potassium, and B vitamins may occur with a low-carb or ketogenic diet.

3. ***Keto Flu***: When transitioning into ketosis, some individuals may experience symptoms such as fatigue, brain fog, and headaches. This is often referred to as the "keto flu" and can last for a few days to a couple of weeks.
4. ***Possible Disruption of Hormonal Balance***: Some research suggests that the ketogenic diet may alter hormone levels in women, potentially impacting menstrual cycles and fertility. More studies are needed in this area.
5. ***Not Suitable for Everyone***: The ketogenic diet may not be suitable for individuals with certain medical conditions or on particular medications. It's essential to consult with a healthcare professional before starting any new dietary approach.

Despite these potential disadvantages, many women over 50 have successfully incorporated the ketogenic diet into their lifestyle and experienced numerous health benefits. As with any dietary change, it's crucial to listen to your body and make adjustments as needed.

It's also essential to focus on nutrient-dense, whole foods and consult with a healthcare professional for personalized recommendations. Ultimately, the ketogenic diet may not be the right fit for everyone, but it can be a valuable tool for those looking to improve their overall health and well-being.

The Types of Ketogenic Diet

The ketogenic diet has several variations, each tailored to suit different needs and lifestyles. Here are the major types of the ketogenic diet:

Standard Ketogenic Diet (SKD)

The Standard Ketogenic Diet (SKD) is the most popular and widely adopted version of the keto diet. This diet involves a significant reduction in carbohydrate intake, restricting carbs to only 5-10% of daily caloric intake. The bulk of the diet, around 70-75%, comes from fats, while the remaining 15-20% is composed of proteins.

To adhere to the SKD, it is recommended to consume foods such as meat, poultry, avocados, butter, and green vegetables. It's crucial to avoid sweet and starchy foods. The allowable amount of carbohydrates should not exceed 50 grams per day. By following these guidelines, individuals can maintain the metabolic state of ketosis and enjoy its benefits.

Targeted Keto Diet (TKD)

The Targeted Keto Diet (TKD) is designed for physically active individuals and athletes who require more carbohydrates to fuel their workouts. Unlike the SKD, the TKD allows for an additional carbohydrate intake of about 70-80 grams per day, on top of the standard 50 grams.

Dietitians often recommend that those following the TKD consume easily digestible carbohydrates found in fruits, dairy products, and whole grains. This approach ensures that the body has enough energy to perform high-intensity exercises while still benefiting from the principles of the ketogenic diet.

Cyclical Keto Diet (CKD)

The Cyclical Keto Diet (CKD) offers a more flexible approach to the ketogenic lifestyle. In CKD, individuals follow the standard ketogenic diet (commonly SKD) for five days a week. On the remaining two days, they can consume non-keto but healthy meals, allowing carbohydrate intake to exceed the usual 50-gram limit.

During these two "carb-loading" days, it is recommended to choose healthy carbohydrate-rich foods like dairy products, fruits, and whole grains, rather than processed or sugary items. This break from strict keto compliance can help alleviate the psychological pressure and stress associated with maintaining a stringent diet, thus promoting better mental health and long-term adherence.

High Protein Keto Diet (HPKD)

The High Protein Keto Diet (HPKD) is a variation that increases protein intake to approximately 30% of daily caloric intake, while still keeping carbohydrates at a maximum of 50 grams per day. This diet is particularly appealing to individuals who prefer to consume more protein-rich foods like meat and poultry, in contrast to the typical fat-dominant standard keto diet.

By increasing protein consumption, the HPKD supports muscle maintenance and growth, making it a suitable option for those who engage in strength training or other forms of resistance exercise. Despite the higher protein allowance, it remains essential to choose healthy fats to ensure overall balance and effectiveness of the diet.

Understanding the different types of ketogenic diets allows individuals to choose the approach that best fits their lifestyle and health goals. Whether one opts for the strict regimen of the Standard Ketogenic Diet, the flexibility of the Cyclical Keto Diet, the targeted support for athletic performance in the Targeted Keto Diet, or the muscle-supporting benefits of the High Protein Keto Diet, each variation offers unique advantages. Consulting with a dietitian or physician can help tailor the diet to meet individual needs, ensuring the best possible outcomes on the ketogenic journey.

How Do You Get Started?

Jumpstarting a keto diet could be a real challenge especially when you are used to consuming many carbohydrates. You can follow this guide to successfully kick-start your keto lifestyle.

Step 1: Do Your Research

Nothing bad comes from being well-informed. Educate yourself first about how the diet works, its effects, and its composition. This foundational knowledge will help you understand the principles behind the ketogenic diet, including how it shifts your body from burning carbohydrates to burning fats for energy. Understanding the science will give you confidence and clarity about what to expect, and how to optimize your diet for the best possible results.

In this digital age, almost all information is at the tip of your fingers. Take advantage of reliable online resources, such as reputable health websites, academic journals, and dietitian blogs. Look for articles, videos, and podcasts that explain the keto diet in detail, covering aspects like macronutrient ratios, meal planning, and potential challenges. Additionally, consider reading books by experts in the field for a comprehensive understanding.

You can also ask friends and relatives who have followed the keto diet about their experiences, opinions, and tips. Personal anecdotes can provide valuable insights that you might not find in scientific literature. These firsthand accounts can help you prepare for common obstacles, offer practical advice on meal preparation, and even recommend specific recipes or food products. Connecting with others who have successfully navigated the keto journey can be both motivating and reassuring.

By combining thorough research with personal testimonials, you'll be well-equipped to start your ketogenic diet journey with confidence. This preparation will enable you to make informed decisions, set realistic goals, and sustain your commitment to the diet.

Step 2: Plan Your Diet Thoroughly

Transitioning from your usual high-carb diet to a low-carb ketogenic diet requires commitment and discipline. The drastic reduction in carbohydrates can be particularly challenging at first, as your body adjusts to using fats instead of carbs for energy.

This initial phase might feel especially draining and even uncomfortable, often referred to as the "keto flu," which includes symptoms like headaches, fatigue, and irritability. However, meticulous planning can help you navigate this transition more smoothly.

1. **Organize Everything Beforehand**

    To ensure your diet goes well, it's crucial to organize every aspect of it in advance. Start by creating detailed meal plans that outline what you'll eat for breakfast, lunch, dinner, and snacks each day. This will help you maintain the correct macronutrient ratios required for a ketogenic diet—typically high fat, moderate protein, and very low carbohydrates.

    Create a shopping list based on your meal plans to ensure you have all the necessary ingredients. Stock up on keto-friendly foods such as avocados, nuts, seeds, olive oil, fatty fish, and leafy greens. Having these supplies on hand will make it easier to stick to your new eating regimen without the temptation of reverting to high-carb options.

2. **Consult Professionals**

    Consider enlisting the help of a dietitian and personal trainer. A dietitian can provide personalized guidance to ensure you're meeting your nutritional needs and help you devise a sustainable meal plan.

They can also monitor your progress and make adjustments as needed. A personal trainer can develop a fitness regimen that complements your dietary changes, helping you build muscle and improve overall health.

3. **Set a Definite Starting Date**

   It's highly encouraged to set a definite starting date for your ketogenic diet. This allows you to mentally prepare for the significant lifestyle change. Use the time leading up to your start date to educate yourself, gather supplies, and gradually reduce your carbohydrate intake to ease the transition. Mental preparedness is critical; being psychologically ready can enhance your commitment and resilience during the initial adjustment period.

4. **Additional Tips for Success**
   - *Stay Hydrated*: Proper hydration can alleviate some symptoms of the keto flu.
   - *Electrolytes*: Incorporate electrolytes into your diet to maintain balance and prevent cramps or fatigue.
   - *Track Progress*: Use apps or journals to monitor your food intake, weight, and any physical changes.
   - *Support System*: Engage with online communities or local support groups for additional encouragement and advice.

By planning your diet thoroughly and preparing both mentally and physically, you'll set yourself up for a successful transition to the ketogenic lifestyle. This thorough preparation will help you remain focused and determined throughout your journey, ultimately increasing your chances of long-term success.

Step 3: Make Your Cupboards and Refrigerator Keto-Friendly

To fully embrace a ketogenic lifestyle, it's essential that your kitchen is just as ready for the transition as you are. A well-prepared kitchen will not only help you stay on track but also make the process more enjoyable and sustainable. By clearing your cupboards and refrigerator of non-keto foods, you minimize the chances of succumbing to high-carb temptations, which can derail your progress toward achieving and maintaining ketosis.

1. **Clear Out Non-Keto Foods**

   Begin by conducting a thorough audit of your kitchen. Remove or donate any foods that are high in carbohydrates, including pasta, bread, rice, sugary snacks, and starchy vegetables. This step is crucial because every time you consume carb-rich foods, you take a step away from ketosis, the metabolic state where your body burns fat for fuel instead of carbohydrates.

2. Stock Up on Keto-Friendly Foods

To ensure you're always prepared to make a keto-friendly meal, stock your kitchen with the following essentials:

- *Meat*: Choose unprocessed meats, preferably grass-fed to ensure higher nutritional quality. Options include beef, pork, lamb, and poultry.
- *Oils*: Healthy fats are a cornerstone of the keto diet. Keep a variety of oils on hand, such as coconut oil and olive oil, which are excellent for cooking and adding to dishes.
- *Vegetables*: Focus on leafy and low-carb vegetables such as spinach, kale, broccoli, cauliflower, zucchini, and asparagus. These provide essential nutrients without adding significant carbs.
- *Fish and Seafood*: Incorporate a variety of fatty fish like salmon, mackerel, and sardines, as well as shellfish like shrimp and crab. These are rich in omega-3 fatty acids, which are beneficial for heart health.
- *Eggs*: A versatile and affordable source of protein and healthy fats, eggs can be used in numerous keto recipes.
- *High-Fat Dairy*: Stock up on butter, heavy cream, and cheese. These add richness to your meals and help you meet your fat intake goals.

- *Non-Sugar Coffee and Tea*: Replace sugar-laden drinks with black coffee or tea. You can add heavy cream or a sugar-free sweetener if desired.
- *Berries*: While most fruits are high in carbs, berries like strawberries, blueberries, raspberries, and blackberries can be enjoyed in moderation.
- *Nuts and Seeds*: Almonds, walnuts, chia seeds, and flaxseeds are excellent for snacking or adding texture to your meals. These nuts and seeds are rich in healthy fats and fiber.

3. **Additional Tips for a Keto-Ready Kitchen:**
- *Organize Your Pantry*: Group keto-friendly items together for easy access. Consider labeling shelves or containers to quickly identify approved foods.
- *Meal Prep*: Prepare and portion out meals ahead of time to avoid last-minute choices that might lead to carb consumption.
- *Recipe Resources*: Keep keto cookbooks or save online recipes to ensure you have plenty of meal ideas that fit your dietary needs.
- *Snack Alternatives*: Keep keto-friendly snacks like cheese sticks, hard-boiled eggs, and nuts readily available to curb hunger and cravings.
- *Stay Educated*: Continue learning about keto-compliant ingredients and new recipes to keep your diet varied and interesting.

By transforming your kitchen into a keto-friendly space, you create an environment that supports your dietary goals and reduces the likelihood of setbacks. This proactive step helps ensure that you have all the tools and ingredients necessary to make delicious, satisfying, and healthful keto meals, reinforcing your commitment to the diet.

Step 4: Equip Yourself with Helpful Tools

The goal of a ketogenic diet is to enter and maintain the state of ketosis, where your body burns fat for fuel instead of carbohydrates. Achieving this metabolic state requires diligent monitoring of your food intake, especially during the initial phases of the diet. To make this process easier and more accurate, equipping yourself with helpful tools is essential.

Calorie-Counting Mobile Apps:

Calorie-counting mobile apps are invaluable for tracking your daily intake of fats, carbs, and proteins. These apps allow you to log each meal, snack, and drink you consume, providing a clear picture of your macronutrient distribution. This is crucial for ensuring you stay within the recommended ratios needed to achieve and sustain ketosis.

Two of the best apps available for this purpose are:

1. *MyFitnessPal*

- Features: MyFitnessPal offers a vast database of foods, including restaurant meals and branded products, making it easy to log your meals accurately. The app also allows you to scan barcodes for quick entry.
- Customization: You can set personalized goals based on your ketogenic diet requirements, adjusting your macronutrient targets accordingly.
- Integration: MyFitnessPal integrates with various fitness trackers, providing a comprehensive view of your calorie expenditure and intake.

2. *MyPlate by Livestrong*
- Features: MyPlate provides a user-friendly interface with a robust food database. It also includes a barcode scanner for easy food logging.
- Guidance: The app offers meal plans and recipes that are tailored to different dietary preferences, including keto.
- Community Support: MyPlate has an active community where you can find support, share experiences, and get tips from other users.

Additional Tools for Success:

Besides mobile apps, consider incorporating other tools to help you stay on track:

- *Digital Food Scale*: A digital food scale helps you measure portion sizes accurately. This precision is

particularly important for foods that contain hidden carbs or fats.
- ***Ketone Meters***: Use a blood ketone meter or breath analyzer to monitor your ketone levels regularly. This helps you determine whether you're in ketosis and adjust your diet as needed.
- ***Meal Prep Containers***: Invest in quality meal prep containers for organizing and storing your meals. This makes it easier to stick to your planned diet and resist impulsive eating.
- ***Recipe Apps and Websites***: Utilize recipe apps and websites dedicated to keto-friendly meals. Having a variety of delicious recipes at your fingertips can keep your diet enjoyable and sustainable.
- ***Kitchen Gadgets***: Consider kitchen gadgets like spiralizers for making zoodles (zucchini noodles) or air fryers for healthier cooking methods that align with keto principles.

Using these tools not only simplifies the process of adhering to a ketogenic diet but also enhances your ability to make informed decisions about what you eat. By consistently tracking your macronutrient intake and monitoring your ketone levels, you can better understand how different foods affect your body and optimize your diet for better results. Additionally, having the right tools at your disposal can reduce stress and increase your confidence in maintaining this lifestyle change.

By equipping yourself with these helpful tools, you set yourself up for success on your ketogenic journey. These resources will help you stay organized, accountable, and motivated as you work towards achieving and sustaining ketosis.

Step 5: Prepare Yourself

Starting a ketogenic diet is a major lifestyle change that can trigger significant reactions from both your mind and body. This transition can be challenging, but understanding and preparing for these challenges will help you successfully navigate them.

1. **Physical and Mental Reactions**

   Your body may initially react negatively to the drastic reduction in carbohydrates. Commonly referred to as the "keto flu," these initial symptoms can include headaches, fatigue, irritability, dizziness, and nausea. These occur as your body adjusts to burning fat for energy instead of carbohydrates. While these symptoms are temporary, they can be uncomfortable and discouraging.

   Similarly, your mind might also struggle with the change. Carbohydrates often provide a quick source of energy and comfort, and their sudden absence can lead to cravings and emotional discomfort. You might experience carb withdrawal symptoms similar to those experienced by individuals quitting smoking or alcohol. This can manifest as mood swings, heightened cravings, and difficulty concentrating.

2. **Emotional and Mental Exhaustion**

Changing your diet can also be emotionally and mentally exhausting. Food is often tied to our social activities, traditions, and comfort mechanisms. Adapting to a new way of eating can feel isolating or overwhelming at times. It's important to acknowledge these feelings as part of the process and develop strategies to cope with them.

Here are some ways to support yourself through this transition:

a. *Mindfulness and Meditation*: Practice mindfulness and meditation to manage stress and stay centered. Simple breathing exercises, guided meditations, or even short mindful moments throughout the day can help keep your mind calm and focused.
b. *Relaxation Techniques*: Engage in relaxation techniques such as yoga, deep breathing exercises, or progressive muscle relaxation to reduce stress levels and promote mental clarity.
c. *Stay Hydrated and Supplement Electrolytes*: Proper hydration can alleviate many symptoms of the keto flu. Drink plenty of water and consider supplementing with

electrolytes like sodium, potassium, and magnesium to maintain balance and prevent dehydration-related discomfort.

d. *Seek Social Support*: Share your journey with friends, family, or online communities who understand and support your goals. Connecting with others who are also following a ketogenic diet can provide encouragement, share tips, and offer valuable insights.

e. *Set Realistic Expectations*: Be patient with yourself and set realistic expectations. Understand that the adjustment period is temporary and that your body will gradually adapt to the new dietary regimen.

f. *Maintain a Balanced Routine*: Ensure you maintain a balanced routine that includes physical activity, adequate sleep, and time for hobbies and relaxation. A well-rounded lifestyle supports both physical and mental health.

g. *Reward Yourself*: Celebrate your progress and milestones along the way. Reward yourself with non-food-related treats like a spa day, a new book, or a relaxing outing. Positive reinforcement can boost your motivation and commitment.

By preparing yourself both physically and mentally, you can better handle the challenges that come with starting a ketogenic diet. Remember that it's normal to face difficulties during such a significant transition. By keeping a healthy mind and body, practicing self-care, and staying committed to your goals, you'll increase your chances of long-term success on your ketogenic journey.

Foods to Eat in the Ketogenic Diet for Women Over 50

For women over 50, following a ketogenic diet can offer numerous health benefits, such as improved metabolic health, weight management, and better energy levels. However, it is essential to focus on nutrient-dense foods that support overall well-being and address age-related nutritional needs. Here's a list of foods to incorporate into a ketogenic diet:

1. **Protein Sources**
- *Fatty Fish*: Salmon, mackerel, sardines, and trout are rich in omega-3 fatty acids, which are beneficial for heart health and inflammation reduction.
- *Grass-Fed Meat*: Beef, lamb, pork, and other meats from grass-fed animals offer higher levels of omega-3 fats and antioxidants.
- *Poultry*: Chicken, turkey, and duck are excellent sources of lean protein.
- *Eggs*: Whole eggs are nutrient-dense and provide high-quality proteins and healthy fats.

Healthy Fats
- *Avocado*: High in monounsaturated fats and fiber, avocados are great for heart health.

- ***Nuts and Seeds***: Almonds, walnuts, chia seeds, flaxseeds, and pumpkin seeds offer a rich source of healthy fats, fiber, and essential minerals.
- ***Oils***: Olive oil, coconut oil, avocado oil, and MCT oil are excellent sources of healthy fats for cooking and dressing salads.
- ***Butter and Ghee***: Preferably grass-fed options, these are rich in healthy fats and can be used in cooking and baking.

Low-Carb Vegetables

- ***Leafy Greens***: Spinach, kale, Swiss chard, and arugula are low in carbs but high in vitamins and minerals.
- ***Cruciferous Vegetables***: Broccoli, cauliflower, Brussels sprouts, and cabbage are versatile and nutrient-packed.
- ***Other Low-Carb Veggies***: Zucchini, bell peppers, asparagus, cucumbers, and mushrooms can be incorporated into various dishes.

Dairy (High-Fat)

- ***Full-Fat Dairy Products***: Cheese, Greek yogurt, heavy cream, and sour cream provide fats and proteins. Opt for full-fat versions without added sugars.
- ***Fermented Dairy***: Kefir and cottage cheese can be beneficial for gut health.

Berries (in moderation)

- *Low-Carb Fruits*: Strawberries, raspberries, blueberries, and blackberries can be enjoyed in small quantities due to their lower carb content compared to other fruits.

Beverages

- *Water*: Staying hydrated is crucial. You can add lemon or lime slices for flavor.
- *Tea and Coffee*: Unsweetened tea and black coffee are keto-friendly. You can add heavy cream or a sugar-free sweetener if desired.
- *Bone Broth*: Rich in nutrients and helpful for electrolyte balance, especially during the initial stages of the diet.

Snacks

- *Cheese Sticks*: Convenient and satisfying high-fat snacks.
- *Hard-Boiled Eggs*: Quick and easy protein-rich snacks.
- *Olives*: A good source of healthy fats and low in carbs.
- *Keto Fat Bombs*: Homemade snacks made with ingredients like coconut oil, nuts, and seeds.

Supplements (If Needed)

- *Electrolytes*: Magnesium, potassium, and sodium supplements can help manage the initial side effects of transitioning to a keto diet, often referred to as the "keto flu."
- *Omega-3 Supplements*: If dietary intake of fatty fish is insufficient, consider an omega-3 supplement.

Foods to Avoid in the Ketogenic Diet for Women Over 50

To maintain ketosis and reap the full benefits of a ketogenic diet, it's essential to avoid foods that are high in carbohydrates and sugars. For women over 50, it's particularly important to steer clear of certain foods that can negatively impact metabolic health, weight management, and overall well-being. Here's a comprehensive list of foods to avoid:

1. **High-Carbohydrate Foods**
- *Grains and Grain Products*: Bread, pasta, rice, oats, quinoa, corn, and barley should be excluded due to their high carbohydrate content.
- *Sugary Foods and Beverages*:
    - *Sugars*: Table sugar, honey, maple syrup, agave nectar, and other sweeteners.
    - *Sweets*: Candy, cookies, cakes, pastries, and ice cream.

- ○ ***Sweetened Beverages***: Soda, fruit juices, sweetened teas, energy drinks, and flavored lattes.

2. **Starchy Vegetables**
- *Potatoes*: White potatoes, sweet potatoes, yams, and other starchy tubers.
- *Corn*: Corn and corn-based products like cornmeal and popcorn.
- *Peas and Legumes*: Beans, lentils, chickpeas, and peanuts (although some nuts and seeds can be eaten in moderation).

3. **Fruits High in Sugar**
- *Tropical Fruits*: Bananas, mangoes, pineapples, and papayas are high in natural sugars.
- *Dried Fruits*: Raisins, dates, figs, and other dried fruits are concentrated sources of sugar.

4. **Processed Foods and Snacks**
- *Chips and Crackers*: Potato chips, tortilla chips, pretzels, and other snack foods made from grains or starches.
- *Baked Goods*: Muffins, bagels, donuts, and other baked items typically made with flour and sugar.
- *Fast Food*: Most fast food items contain hidden sugars, unhealthy fats, and carbohydrates.

5. **Dairy with Added Sugars and Low-Fat Options**
- *Flavored Yogurts*: Often contain added sugars; opt for plain, full-fat versions instead.

- *Low-Fat Dairy Products*: These often have higher sugar content to compensate for reduced fat.

6. **Sugary Condiments and Sauces**
- *Ketchup*: Contains added sugars.
- *Barbecue Sauce*: Many commercial versions are high in sugars.
- *Salad Dressings*: Many store-bought dressings have added sugars; choose homemade or sugar-free options.

7. **Unhealthy Fats and Oils**
- *Trans Fats*: Avoid partially hydrogenated oils found in many processed foods.
- *Refined Oils*: Limit intake of vegetable oils such as soybean oil, corn oil, and sunflower oil, which can cause inflammation.

8. **Alcoholic Beverages**
- *Beer*: High in carbs and should be avoided.
- *Sweet Wines and Cocktails*: Contain added sugars and syrups.

By avoiding or limiting these foods, you can reduce your sugar intake and improve your overall health. Instead, opt for whole, unprocessed foods like fruits, vegetables, lean proteins, and healthy fats. These foods provide essential nutrients and are lower in added sugars.

Favorite Keto Meal Plans and Recipes

7-Day Sample Meal Plan

Below is a sample 7-day meal plan to give you an idea of how to incorporate low-carb, high-protein meals into your week. Keep in mind that this is just one example and you can mix and match recipes to fit your preferences and dietary needs.

Day 1

Breakfast: Western Omelet

Lunch:

Sesame Chicken with a side of Roasted Veggies

Dinner:

Baked Turkey Wings with a serving of Cauliflower Mash

Day 2

Breakfast: Mushroom Omelet

Lunch: Keto Pesto Chicken with a side salad (mixed greens, cucumber, avocado)

Dinner: Grilled Lamb with sautéed spinach and garlic

Day 3

Breakfast: Zero Carb Bread with avocado and poached eggs

Lunch: Ground Beef Stroganoff with zucchini noodles

Dinner: Mexican Style Beef Chili with cauliflower rice

Day 4

Breakfast: Bacon and Eggs

Lunch: Steak and Mushrooms with a side of steamed broccoli

Dinner: Zero Carb Buttery Noodles with shrimp scampi

Day 5

Breakfast: Greek Yogurt with berries and chia seeds

Lunch: Chicken Caesar Salad (grilled chicken, romaine lettuce, parmesan, Caesar dressing)

Dinner: Cauliflower Pizza topped with pepperoni, mozzarella, and fresh basil

Day 6

Breakfast: Keto Smoothie (spinach, avocado, almond milk, protein powder)

Lunch: Sesame Ginger Salmon with a side of roasted Brussels sprouts

Dinner: Pulled Pork with coleslaw

Day 7

Breakfast: Almond Flour Pancakes with a side of bacon

Lunch: Tuna Salad Lettuce Wraps (tuna, mayonnaise, celery, wrapped in large lettuce leaves)

Dinner: Grilled Chicken Thighs with asparagus

Snacks (Optional)

- Cheese sticks
- Hard-boiled eggs
- Nuts and seeds
- Avocado slices
- Olives

Desserts (Optional)

- Keto fat bombs (cream cheese, butter, stevia, cocoa powder)
- Chia seed pudding (chia seeds, unsweetened almond milk, vanilla extract)

By varying your meals each day and incorporating different recipes, you can enjoy a diverse and satisfying ketogenic diet tailored to women over 50.

Sample Recipes

These are some of the top keto meals loved by all types of palates.

Cauliflower Pizza

Ingredients:

- cauliflower
- 1/4 cup of tomato pasta sauce
- 1/4 cup of pesto sauce (no sugar)
- 100 grams of thinly sliced mozzarella
- 250 grams of cut tomatoes
- 2-3 medium-sized eggs
- basil leaves

Instructions:

Cauliflower-made dough

1. Wash the cauliflower.
2. Roughly chop the washed vegetables.
3. Place the chopped cauliflower into a food processor and pulse until fine-looking.
4. Squeeze any remnants of water from the processed cauliflower
5. Spread the dough over baking trays lined with baking paper.
6. Bake the cauliflower dough for 15 minutes in an oven preheated to 140 C.
7. Let the dough sit and cool down.
8. Place the baked cauliflower in the food processor, with almond meal, oil, parmesan, a pinch of salt and peppers, and eggs.

9. Whiz until smooth.
10. Spread the cauliflower dough in a circular shape on the same pan.
11. Roast at 180°C for 25 minutes.
12. Once done, let it cool for a couple of minutes.
13. Start spreading tomato sauce and half of the pesto sauce.
14. Top it with the mozzarella cheese and then bake it at 250°C for 5-10 minutes until the cheese is melted.
15. While waiting, mix the tomato with the remaining pesto sauce.
16. Put tomatoes and basil on top of the freshly baked pizza.
17. Serve and enjoy while warm.

Steak and Mushrooms

Ingredients:

- 4 T-bone beef steak
- 1/4 cup rice bran oil
- 600 grams of Asian mushrooms (e.g. Shiitake, Oyster, Swiss Brown, King Brown)
- 1 cup coriander
- 1 cup mint leaves
- 1/4 garlic chives
- 4 celery sticks
- 2 carrots, thinly sliced
- 200 grams of sugar snaps
- 1/4 red onion, thinly sliced

For the dressing:

- 1/4 cup soy sauce
- 1/4 cup mirin
- 2 tbsp. rice vinegar
- 1 long red chili, finely chopped
- 2 tsp. grated gingers
- 1 crushed garlic clove

Instructions:

Dressing:

1. Put the ingredients of the dressing together in a screw-cap glass jar.

2. Seal the jar and shake well to combine.

T-bone Steak:

1. Heat a barbecue or grilling pan.
2. Place the steaks over the grills.
3. Brush the steaks with oil. Season the meat with herbs, salt, and pepper.
4. For medium-rare, cook each side for about 6 minutes.
5. Place the mushrooms on the grilling pan, brush with oil, and allow to cook well.
6. Combine the cooked mushrooms with the prepared dressing sauce.
7. While waiting for the meat to cook, mix carrots, snaps, and red onion in a bowl to make a salad. Add some dressing.
8. Place the steak on a plate topped with mushrooms and garlic chives.
9. Serve with salad and the remaining dressing.

Ketogenic Pizza

Ingredients:

Crust:

- 4 eggs
- 6 oz. shredded cheese, mozzarella, or provolone

Toppings:

- 1 tsp. dried oregano
- 3 tbsp. unsweetened tomato sauce
- 1-1/2 oz. pepperoni
- 5 oz. shredded cheese
- optional: olives optional

Salad:

- 4 tbsp. olive oil
- 2 oz. leafy greens
- ground black pepper
- sea salt

Instructions:

1. Prepare the oven by preheating to 400°F.
2. Stir eggs and shredded cheese into a medium-sized bowl.
3. Transfer the batter to a baking sheet with parchment paper.
4. Bake until the crust turns golden, about 15 minutes.

5. Once done, take it out and leave to cool for 1-2 minutes.
6. Adjust the temperature of the oven to about 450°F.
7. On the crust, put tomato sauce and sprinkle oregano.
8. Add cheese, followed by pepperoni and olives.
9. Bake in the oven for about 5-10 minutes.
10. Toss the ingredients of the salad.
11. Serve immediately.

Keto Pesto Chicken

Ingredients:

- 1-1/2 lbs chicken thighs breasts, boneless and cut into bite-sized pieces
- pepper
- salt
- 2 tbsp. butter or coconut oil
- 5 tbsp. red or green pesto
- 1-1/4 cups heavy whipping cream
- 5 oz. feta cheese, diced
- 3 oz. pitted olives
- 1 garlic clove, finely chopped

Salad:

- 5 oz. leafy greens
- 4 tbsp. olive oil
- sea salt
- ground black pepper

Instructions:

1. Preheat the oven to 400°F.
2. Season the chicken with salt and pepper.
3. Add butter or oil to a large skillet. Fry the chicken pieces on medium-high heat until golden brown.
4. In a bowl, combine heavy cream and pesto. Mix well.

5. Put the fried chicken meat in a baking dish. Add in olives, garlic, and feta cheese.
6. Pour the pesto or cream mixture.
7. Bake in the oven for 20-30 minutes.
8. Toss all the salad ingredients upon serving.
9. Serve and enjoy.

Mushroom Omelet

Ingredients:

- 3 eggs
- 1 oz. butter, for frying
- 1 oz. shredded cheese
- 1/4 yellow onion, chopped
- 4 large mushrooms, sliced
- salt
- pepper

Instructions:

1. Crack the eggs into a mixing bowl. Beat well with a fork.
2. In a skillet, melt butter on medium heat.
3. Add onion and mushrooms to the skillet. Saute for about 5 minutes until they are soft.
4. Pour in beaten eggs, making sure to evenly spread across the skillet.
5. Let the omelet cook for about 2-3 minutes or until it starts to set around the edges.
6. Sprinkle shredded cheese over one side of the omelet.
7. Fold the other half over the cheese and press down gently with a spatula to seal.
8. Cook for an additional minute or until the cheese is melted and the filling is heated through.
9. Slide the omelet onto a plate and serve hot.

Sesame Chicken

Ingredients:

Coating & Chicken:

- 1 egg
- 1 lb. chicken thighs, cut into bite-sized pieces
- 1 tbsp. arrowroot powder
- 1 tbsp. toasted sesame seed oil
- salt
- pepper

Sesame Sauce:

- 1 tbsp. toasted sesame seed oil
- 1 tbsp. vinegar
- 2 tbsp. soy sauce
- ginger cubed into 1 cm
- 2 tbsp. Sukrin Gold
- 2 tbsp. sesame seeds
- 1/4 tsp. xanthan gum
- 1 clove garlic

Instructions:

1. In a mixing bowl, crack the egg and beat well.
2. Add in arrowroot powder, toasted sesame seed oil, salt, and pepper to the beaten egg. Mix until well combined.
3. Coat the chicken pieces with this mixture.
4. Heat oil in a skillet over medium-high heat.

5. Once hot, add chicken pieces to the skillet and cook for about 6-8 minutes on each side or until they are cooked through.
6. While the chicken is cooking, prepare the sesame sauce by combining toasted sesame seed oil, vinegar, soy sauce, ginger cubes, Sukrin Gold, sesame seeds, xanthan gum, and garlic clove in a small pot over medium heat.
7. Let it simmer for about 5 minutes or until the sauce thickens.
8. Once the chicken is cooked, remove it from the heat and pour the sesame sauce over it.
9. Toss the chicken well in the sauce until all pieces are coated.
10. Serve hot with your choice of rice or vegetables on the side.

Mexican Style Beef Chili

Ingredients:

- 1/2 red pepper, diced
- 1 lb. ground beef
- 3 tbsp. taco seasoning
- 1/4 onion, diced
- 12 oz. fresh or frozen cauliflower rice
- 1 cup tomatoes, diced
- 1-1/2 cups shredded Cheddar cheese or Mexican Blend
- 1/2 cup chicken broth

Instructions:

1. In a large skillet, cook the ground beef over medium heat until it is browned.
2. Add the diced red pepper and onion to the skillet and continue cooking for another 3-4 minutes.
3. Sprinkle taco seasoning over the mixture and stir well.
4. Pour in chicken broth and add cauliflower rice to the skillet.
5. Stir everything together until combined, then let it simmer for about 8-10 minutes or until the cauliflower rice is cooked through.
6. Once done, remove from heat and top with diced tomatoes and shredded cheese.
7. Cover the skillet with a lid and let it sit for about 5 minutes or until the cheese is melted.

8. Serve hot as a delicious low-carb alternative to traditional beef chili.
9. If desired, you can also top it with some fresh cilantro and a dollop of sour cream for added flavor.

Western Omelet

Ingredients:

- 6 eggs
- 2 tbsp. sour cream or heavy whipping cream
- salt
- pepper
- 3 oz. shredded cheese
- 2 oz. butter
- 1/2 yellow onion, chopped finely
- 5 oz. ham, smoked deli, diced
- 1/2 green bell pepper, chopped finely

Instructions:

1. In a small bowl, beat together the eggs, sour cream or heavy whipping cream, and a pinch of salt and pepper.
2. Heat butter in a large skillet over medium heat until sizzling.
3. Add the chopped onion and green bell pepper to the skillet and cook for about 3-4 minutes until softened.
4. Pour the beaten egg mixture into the skillet with the vegetables.
5. Spread diced ham over one-half of the omelet after it begins to set.
6. Sprinkle shredded cheese over the top evenly, then fold over the other half of the omelet on top of the filling.

7. Cook for an additional 2-3 minutes or until the eggs are cooked through and the cheese is melted.
8. Serve hot as a delicious and hearty breakfast option.

For added flavor, you can also add in some diced tomatoes or top with avocado slices before serving. Enjoy your homemade western omelet!

Grilled Lamb

Ingredients:

- 1-1/2 lb. baby spinach leaves
- 3 tbsp. dried oregano, chopped
- 1/4 cup lemon juice
- 1/4 cup olive oil
- 2 tbsp. ground cumin
- 1 tsp. crushed red pepper
- 1 tbsp. coarse sea salt
- 1 tbsp. squeezed juice from an orange
- 3 cloves garlic
- 2 yellow onions, chopped
- cooking spray

Instructions:

1. Begin by preparing the marinade for the lamb. In a large bowl, mix together the lemon juice, olive oil, dried oregano, ground cumin, crushed red pepper, coarse sea salt, and squeezed orange juice.
2. Peel and crush 3 cloves of garlic and add them to the marinade mixture.
3. Place the lamb in a large resealable plastic bag and pour the marinade over it.
4. Seal the bag tightly and massage the marinade into the meat until it is well coated.

5. Refrigerate for at least 4 hours or overnight to allow the flavors to fully infuse into the lamb.
6. Preheat your grill to high heat.
7. Remove lamb from the marinade and discard excess marinade. Thread the meat onto skewers, alternating with chopped onions.
8. Spray cooking spray onto the grill to prevent sticking. Place skewers on the grill and cook for 10-15 minutes, turning occasionally to ensure even cooking.
9. Once cooked to desired doneness, remove from heat and let rest for a few minutes before serving.
10. Serve with a side of grilled vegetables or rice pilaf for a complete meal. Enjoy your delicious and flavorful grilled lamb!

Roasted Veggies

Ingredients:

- 1/2 lb. turnips
- 1/2 lb. carrots
- 1/2 lb. parsnips
- 2 shallots, peeled
- 1/4 tsp. ground black pepper
- 1 tbsp. extra-virgin olive oil
- 6 cloves garlic
- 3/4 tsp. kosher salt
- 2 tbsp. fresh rosemary needles

Instructions:

1. Preheat the oven to 425°F.
2. Wash and peel the turnips, carrots, and parsnips. Cut them into small chunks or cubes.
3. In a large bowl, mix the chopped veggies with the peeled shallots.
4. Add in ground black pepper and drizzle with extra-virgin olive oil, tossing until well coated.
5. Transfer the veggies onto a baking sheet lined with parchment paper or foil.
6. Peel and crush 6 cloves of garlic and add them on top of the vegetables.
7. Sprinkle kosher salt over everything and scatter fresh rosemary needles on top.

8. Roast for 25-30 minutes, stirring occasionally to ensure even cooking.
9. Once tender and lightly browned, remove from the oven and let cool for a few minutes before serving.

Ground Beef Stroganoff

Ingredients:

- 1 lb. 80% lean ground beef
- 2 tbsp. butter
- 1 clove garlic, minced
- 10 oz. sliced mushrooms
- 1 tbsp. fresh parsley, chopped
- 1 tbsp. fresh lemon juice
- salt
- pepper
- 2 tbsp. water

Instructions:

1. In a large skillet, melt the butter over medium heat.
2. Add in minced garlic and sauté for 1 minute until fragrant.
3. Increase the heat to medium-high and add ground beef to the pan. Cook until browned, breaking it up into small pieces as it cooks.
4. Once fully cooked, drain any excess fat from the pan.
5. Return the skillet to medium heat and add sliced mushrooms, stirring occasionally until they become tender.

6. Season with salt and pepper to taste.
7. Stir in chopped fresh parsley and lemon juice, then simmer for an additional 5 minutes.
8. If desired, you can also add 2 tablespoons of water or beef broth to create a creamier sauce consistency.

Banana Bread

Ingredients:

- 1 cup olive oil mayonnaise
- 2 eggs
- 4 medium ripe bananas, mashed
- 2 tsp. vanilla extract
- 2 cups unbleached all-purpose flour
- 1 cup whole wheat flour
- 3/4 cup Brown Xylitol
- 2 tsp. baking soda
- 2 tsp. sea salt
- 2 tsp. cinnamon
- 1 tsp. baking powder
- Optional: flax, nuts, wheat germ, or whey protein

Instructions:

1. Preheat the oven to 350°F.
2. In a large mixing bowl, combine olive oil mayonnaise, eggs, mashed bananas, and vanilla extract. Mix until well combined.
3. In a separate bowl, whisk together the all-purpose flour, whole wheat flour, Brown Xylitol, baking soda, sea salt, cinnamon, and baking powder.
4. Slowly add the dry mixture to the wet mixture while stirring until well combined.

5. If desired, you can also mix in additional ingredients such as flax seeds, nuts, wheat germ, or whey protein for added nutrition and flavor.
6. Grease a 9x5 inch loaf pan with cooking spray or butter.
7. Pour batter into pan and spread evenly.
8. Bake for 50-60 minutes, or until a toothpick inserted in the center comes out clean.
9. Let cool for 10 minutes before removing from pan and slicing to serve.
10. Serve warm or at room temperature with butter or your favorite spread.

Zero Carb Buttery Noodles

Ingredients:

- 7 oz. shirataki noodles
- 2 tbsp. unsalted butter
- 1 tbsp. grated parmesan
- salt
- black pepper
- fresh basil or parsley

Instructions:

1. Drain and rinse shirataki noodles in a colander.
2. In a large saucepan, melt butter over medium heat.
3. Add shirataki noodles to the pan and cook for 3-4 minutes, stirring occasionally.
4. Remove from heat and sprinkle grated parmesan over the noodles.
5. Season with salt and black pepper to taste.
6. Garnish with fresh basil or parsley if desired.
7. Serve hot as a side dish or mix in protein of choice for a complete meal.
8. Enjoy the guilt-free pleasure of eating delicious noodles without any carbs!

Zero Carb Bread

Ingredients:

- 3 eggs
- 3 tbsp. cream cheese at room temperature
- 1/4 tsp. baking powder

Instructions:

1. Preheat oven to 375°F.
2. Separate egg whites from yolks and place them in separate bowls.
3. In the bowl with egg yolks, add cream cheese and baking powder. Mix until well combined.
4. In the bowl with egg whites, beat until stiff peaks form.
5. Gently fold the egg white mixture into the yolk mixture, being careful not to deflate the egg whites too much.
6. Pour batter into a greased 8x4 inch loaf pan.
7. Bake for 25-30 minutes or until golden brown on top and the toothpick inserted in the center comes out clean.
8. Let cool for 10 minutes before removing from pan and slicing to serve as bread slices.

Baked Turkey Wings

Ingredients:

- 4 pcs. or about 5 lbs. whole turkey wings
- 1 tbsp. olive oil
- salt
- pepper
- 1 tsp. paprika

Instructions:

1. Preheat oven to 375°F.
2. Rinse turkey wings and pat dry with paper towels.
3. Place turkey wings in a large baking dish or roasting pan.
4. Drizzle olive oil over the wings and rub to coat them evenly.
5. Season with salt, pepper, and paprika on both sides of the wings.
6. Bake for 1 hour and 30 minutes, flipping the wings halfway through cooking time.
7. Wings are done when they reach an internal temperature of 165°F and are golden brown and crispy on the outside.
8. Let cool for a few minutes before serving with your favorite side dishes like roasted vegetables or cauliflower mash.

Enjoy a low-carb alternative to traditional Thanksgiving turkey without sacrificing flavor or satisfaction. You can also use this recipe for any other occasion and customize the seasonings to your liking.

Conclusion

Thank you for taking the time to read through this comprehensive guide on the ketogenic diet for women over 50. We hope it has been both informative and inspiring, providing you with the knowledge and confidence to start or continue your keto journey.

The ketogenic diet is more than just a popular trend—it's a healthy lifestyle change that emphasizes high-fat, low-carb foods. By helping your body enter a state called ketosis, the ketogenic diet allows you to burn fat for fuel instead of carbohydrates. This can lead to numerous health benefits, especially for women over 50.

One of the primary reasons many people turn to the ketogenic diet is for weight management. Reducing your carb intake and increasing your fat consumption can make it easier to shed excess pounds. Additionally, many followers of the ketogenic diet report higher energy levels and improved stamina, which can be particularly beneficial as you age. It helps you stay active and engaged in your daily activities.

Another common benefit is enhanced mental clarity and focus. The brain thrives on ketones (the byproducts of fat breakdown), leading many people to feel more alert and less foggy when following a ketogenic diet. Furthermore, the ketogenic diet can help stabilize blood sugar levels, which is crucial for preventing and managing type 2 diabetes—a condition that becomes more common with age.

Starting any new diet can be daunting, but with the right mindset and approach, you can achieve your goals. Consistency is crucial. Stick to your meal plans, monitor your carb intake, and remember why you started this journey in the first place. Small, consistent efforts will lead to significant results over time.

Listen to your body because everyone's body reacts differently to dietary changes. Pay attention to how you feel, and make adjustments as necessary. If something doesn't feel right, don't hesitate to tweak your diet or seek advice from a healthcare professional. Drinking plenty of water is essential to the ketogenic diet. It helps prevent dehydration and can reduce symptoms like headaches and fatigue. Aim to drink at least eight glasses of water a day.

Having a support system can make a world of difference. Join a local or online keto community, share your experiences, and learn from others who are on the same path. Support and encouragement from others can help you stay motivated. Finally, results may not come overnight, and that's perfectly okay. Celebrate your progress, no matter how small. Remember, lasting change takes time, and you're building habits that will benefit your long-term health.

To help you along the way, here are some practical tips for making the ketogenic diet work for you.

Meal planning can save you time and ensure you always have keto-friendly options available. Prepare your meals in advance, and always have healthy snacks on hand to avoid temptation. You don't need to make elaborate meals to succeed on the keto diet. Simple recipes with whole, unprocessed foods can be just as effective. Focus on quality ingredients and cooking methods that you enjoy.

Keeping a food diary or using a mobile app to track your carb intake can help you stay accountable and see your progress over time. It can also help you identify any areas where you might need to adjust. Continue to learn about the ketogenic diet and how it affects your body. The more you know, the better equipped you'll be to make informed decisions about your health. Remember, this is a lifestyle change, not a quick fix. Enjoy the process, experiment with new recipes, and find joy in taking care of your health.

Embarking on a ketogenic diet after 50 can be a transformative experience. It's not just about losing weight; it's about gaining energy, improving your mental clarity, and feeling better overall. The journey may have its ups and downs, but your commitment to better health is what truly matters.

Thank you once again for reading this guide. We hope it has empowered you with the knowledge and confidence to start or continue your ketogenic diet journey. Remember, every step you take towards better health is a victory. Stay committed, stay informed, and most importantly, be kind to yourself. Here's to your health and happiness!

FAQs for the Ketogenic Diet for Women Over 50

What is the ketogenic diet and how does it work?

The ketogenic diet is a high-fat, low-carbohydrate eating plan that aims to put your body into a state called ketosis. In ketosis, your body burns fat for fuel instead of carbohydrates. This shift can help with weight management, improve energy levels, and enhance mental clarity. The diet typically involves consuming around 70-75% of your daily calories from fats, 20-25% from proteins, and only about 5-10% from carbohydrates.

Is the ketogenic diet safe for women over 50?

For many women over 50, the ketogenic diet can be safe and beneficial, but it's important to consult with your healthcare provider before starting any new diet plan. Factors such as pre-existing medical conditions, medications, and individual health goals should all be considered. Your doctor can provide personalized advice and help you monitor your progress to ensure the diet is working well for you.

How can the ketogenic diet help with menopause symptoms?

The ketogenic diet may help alleviate some menopause symptoms by stabilizing blood sugar levels and reducing inflammation. Many women report fewer hot flashes, better sleep, and improved mood when following a ketogenic diet. Additionally, the diet's emphasis on healthy fats can support hormone production, which may also help balance hormone-related issues during menopause.

Will I need to take supplements while on the ketogenic diet?

While a well-balanced ketogenic diet can provide most of the nutrients you need, some supplements might be beneficial. Common supplements for those on a ketogenic diet include electrolytes (such as sodium, potassium, and magnesium), vitamin D, omega-3 fatty acids, and fiber. Again, it's best to consult with your healthcare provider to determine which supplements, if any, are appropriate for you.

How quickly can I expect to see results on the ketogenic diet?

The time it takes to see results on the ketogenic diet can vary from person to person. Some individuals notice changes in their energy levels and mental clarity within a few days, while weight loss and other health benefits may take a few weeks to become apparent. Consistency is key, so sticking to the diet and monitoring your progress regularly will help you achieve the best results.

Can I exercise while following the ketogenic diet?

Yes, you can and should exercise while following the ketogenic diet. Physical activity is an important part of a healthy lifestyle and can help enhance the benefits of the keto diet. Initially, you might experience a temporary dip in energy as your body adjusts to using fat for fuel. However, many people find that their energy levels improve and stabilize once they are fully adapted to ketosis. Low-impact exercises like walking, yoga, and swimming can be especially beneficial.

What are common challenges when starting the ketogenic diet, and how can I overcome them?

Common challenges when starting the ketogenic diet include the "keto flu," cravings for high-carb foods, and difficulty maintaining social eating habits. The keto flu, characterized by symptoms like headaches, fatigue, and irritability, usually lasts for a few days to a week and can be mitigated by staying hydrated and replenishing electrolytes. To manage cravings, focus on eating satisfying, nutrient-dense keto-friendly foods. Planning and preparing meals in advance can help you stay on track. For social situations, consider bringing your own keto-friendly dishes or researching restaurant menus ahead of time to find suitable options.

References

Harvard Health. (2022b, August 9). Ketogenic diet: Is the ultimate low-carb diet good for you? https://www.health.harvard.edu/blog/ketogenic-diet-is-the-ultimate-low-carb-diet-good-for-you-2017072712089

University of Southern California. (2023, September 19). Fad diets could contribute to liver disease known as a 'silent killer' USC Today. https://today.usc.edu/fad-diets-keto-nonalcoholic-fatty-liver-disease/

Gill, L. E., Bartels, S. J., & Batsis, J. A. (2015). Weight management in older adults. Current Obesity Reports, 4(3), 379–388. https://doi.org/10.1007/s13679-015-0161-z

Helms, N. (n.d.). Ketogenic diet: What are the risks? https://www.uchicagomedicine.org/forefront/health-and-wellness-articles/ketogenic-diet-what-are-the-risks

Kapoor, E., Collazo-Clavell, M. L., & Faubion, S. S. (2017). Weight Gain in Women at Midlife: A Concise Review of the Pathophysiology and Strategies for Management. Mayo Clinic Proceedings, 92(10), 1552–1558. https://doi.org/10.1016/j.mayocp.2017.08.004

Paoli, A., Rubini, A., Volek, J. S., & Grimaldi, K. A. (2013). Beyond weight loss: a review of the therapeutic uses of very-low-carbohydrate (ketogenic) diets. European Journal of Clinical Nutrition, 67(8), 789–796. https://doi.org/10.1038/ejcn.2013.116

Stacey, D., Jull, J., Beach, S., Dumas, A., Strychar, I., Adamo, K., Brochu, M., & Prud'homme, D. (2015). Middle-aged women's decisions about body weight management. Menopause, 22(4), 414–422. https://doi.org/10.1097/gme.0000000000000326

www.ingramcontent.com/pod-product-compliance
Lightning Source LLC
LaVergne TN
LVHW012033060526
838201LV00061B/4592